Contents

Preface..2
Reception..5
Anamnesis...11
Massage...23
Manual therapy..28
PNF..38
Mulligan...43
Exercises...46
Gait training..53
Lymphatic drainage...55
Electrotherapy...59
pelvic floor exercises..62
Breathing therapy...66
Useful..69
Thanks..71
Bibliography..72

Preface

Who am I?

My name is Caroline Braun and I created the Little Physio.
I studied translation and worked as a freelance translator.
I then decided to change my way of living and became a physical therapist / physiotherapist.
I've been working as a physical therapist for over 10 years in different hospitals as well as in private practices.

Why did I create Little Physio?

My experience has shown me the difficulties of treating patients who don't speak the same language.
It's difficult and even sometimes impossible to diagnose or treat the patient correctly.
The consequences for the patient are disastrous.

Many people think that the patient has to speak the language of the country he or she lives in.
Even if correct it's also not always possible.
Some people are not able to learn or have just arrived.
Others might be on vacation or are only here temporarily to work.

I am a physical therapist and my job is not to judge but to treat the patients.
And I have to treat them the best I can.

That's why I created "Little Physio".

This translator enables the therapist to communicate and to treat foreign patients.

Your therapy will become easier and better.

The book is divided into 14 chapters like "Reception", "Massage", "Manual therapy", "Exercises" and so on. This makes it easier and faster for you to find the sentences you need.

In addition to the book, you have the opportunity to get the **Little Physio App for mobile phones and tabs, iphone and ipad.**

The Apps are available on the Apple Appstore and on the Googleplaystore.

The **Little Physio Apps are the audio version of the books**.

It is as easy as clicking on the needed sentence and your cell phone or tab "speaks" it out in the foreign language.

You can see a demo on:

littlephysio.com

or on

youtube

I became a physical therapist to help others, no matter if they speak my language or not.

Now, it is possible!

Reception

Empfang

1. Hello
Guten Tag

2. My name is
Ich heiße...

3. Do you have a doctor's prescription?
Haben Sie ein Rezept vom Arzt?

4. Yes
JA

5. No
NEIN

6. Do you have your insurance card?
Haben Sie Ihre Versicherungskarte?

7. Would you please bring the insurance card next time?

Können Sie das nächste mal die Karte bringen?

8. Would you please write down your phone number?

Können Sie mir bitte Ihre Telefonnummer aufschreiben?

9. There is a mistake in the prescription. You have to go back to your doctor and have him issue a new one.

Da ist ein Fehler beim Rezept, Sie müssen wieder zum Arzt damit er Ihnen ein neues Rezept gibt.

10. Do you have a report / X-ray / CT- images from your doctor?

Haben Sie einen Bericht / Röntgen, CT-Bilder vom Arzt?

11. Would you please bring the x-rays / the report with you next time?

Können Sie das nächste Mal die Bilder, den Bericht mitnehmen?

12. Here are your appointments

Da sind Ihre Termine

13. If these appointments don't work for you, please let me know.

Wenn die Termine für Sie nicht gehen, sagen Sie es mir.

14. This one doesn't work?

Da geht es nicht?

15. Not on this day at all?

An dem Tag nicht?

16. Rather in the morning?

Lieber Vormittags

17. Rather in the afternoon?

Lieber Nachmittags

18. Monday

Montag

19. Tuesday

Dienstag

20. Wednesday
Mittwoch

21. Thursday
Donnerstag

22. Friday
Freitag

23. Saturday
Samstag

24. Sunday
Sonntag

25. I'm sorry, you are too early
Es tut mir Leid, Sie sind zu früh

26. I'm sorry, you are too late
Es tut mir Leid, Sie sind zu spät

27. This week won't work
Diese Woche geht es nicht

28. Today doesn't work
Heute geht es nicht

29. Not before next week
Erst nächste Woche

30. Not before next month
Erst nächsten Monat

31. The therapist is on vacation
Die Therapeutin / der Therapeut ist in Urlaub

32. The therapist is ill
Die Therapeutin / der Therapeut ist krank

33. Would you like to work with a different therapist?
Wollen Sie zum anderen Therapeut ?

34. Yes
JA

35. No
NEIN

36. Would you like to continue with the same therapist?

Wollen Sie bei demselben Therapeut / derselben Therapeutin bleiben?

37. Would you rather wait until your therapist is back?

Wollen sie warten bis der Therapeut / die Therapeutin wieder da ist?

38. Here is your bill.

Hier ist Ihre Rechnung.

39. Would you like to pay now?

Wollen Sie jetzt Zahlen?

40. Do you want to pay cash?

Wollen Sie bar zahlen?

Anamnesis

Anamnese

1. Please undress

Ziehen Sie sich aus bitte

2. Can you please take off your top ?

Können Sie Ihr Oberteil ausziehen?

3. Can you please take off your pants?

Können Sie Ihre Hose ausziehen?

4. Can you please take off your skirt?

Können Sie ihren Rock ausziehen?

5. Are you in pain?

Haben Sie Schmerzen?

6. Yes

Ja

7. No
Nein

8. Show me where it hurts
Zeigen Sie mir wo Sie Schmerzen haben

9. Where does it hurt?
Wo haben Sie Schmerzen?

10. Is the pain radiating into your arm?
Strahlen Sie in den Arm aus?

11. Is the pain radiating into your leg?
Strahlen Sie in das Bein aus?

12. Where does the pain radiate into?
Bis wohin strahlen die Schmerzen?

13. Show me
Zeigen Sie es mir

14. Do you feel numbness?
Haben Sie Taubheitsgefühle?

15. Where?
Wo?

16. Do you have paralytic symptoms?
Haben Sie Lähmungserscheinungen?

17. Do you feel formication?
Haben Sie Ameisenlaufen?

18. Where?
Wo?

19. When did it start?
Seit wann?

20. For days
Seit Tagen

21. For weeks
Seit Wochen

22. For months
Seit Monaten

23. For years
Seit Jahren

24. What does the pain feel like?
Wie ist der Schmerz?

25. Acute
Stechend

26. Dull
Dumpf

27. Dragging
Ziehend

28. Did the pain develop slowly?

Ist der Schmerz langsam entstanden?

29. Did the pain develop fast?

Ist der Schmerz schnell entstanden?

30. Does the pain last for a long time?

Hält der Schmerz lange?

31. Several seconds

Mehrere Sekunden

32. Several minutes

Mehrere Minuten

33. Several hours

Mehrere Stunden

34. Several days

Mehrere Tage

35. Did you have an accident?

Hatten Sie einen Unfall?

36. Have you had treatment yet?

Sind Sie schon behandelt worden?

37. Yes

Ja

38. No

Nein

39. Do you have high blood pressure?

Haben sie Bluthochdruck?

40. Do you have diabetes?

Haben Sie Diabetis?

41. Are you dizzy?

Ist Ihnen schwindelig?

42. Are you pregnant?

Sind Sie schwanger?

43. What month?

Im wievielten Monat?

44. Do you take pain killers?

Nehmen Sie Schmerzmittel?

45. Do you take blood thinning medication?

Nehmen Sie Blutverdünnungsmedikamente / Medikamente ?

46. Do you have problems with your thyroid?

Haben Sie Probleme mit der Schilddrüse?

47. Do you have heart problems?

Haben Sie Herzprobleme?

48. Do you have a headache?

Haben Sie Kopfschmerzen?

49. Did you have surgery?
Sind Sie operiert worden?

50. When did you have surgery?
Wann sind Sie operiert worden?

51. A few days ago
Vor Tagen

52. A few months ago
Vor Monaten

53. A few years ago
Vor Jahren

54. You have to see a doctor.
Sie müssen zum Arzt gehen

55. Does it hurt when you are moving?
Haben Sie Schmerzen bei Belastung?

56. Do you have pain while resting?

Haben Sie Ruheschmerzen?

57. When does it hurt most? When is the pain worst?

Wann sind die Schmerzen am schlimmsten?

58. In the morning

Morgens

59. In the evening

Abends

60. At night

Nachts

61. Always the same

Immer gleich

62. While going up

Beim Gehen aufwärts

63. While going down

Beim Gehen abwärts

64. Going up the stairs

Beim Treppenhochsteigen

65. Going down the stairs

Beim Treppenruntersteigen

66. While sitting for a long time

Beim langen Sitzen?

67. After sitting for a long time

Nach langem Sitzen?

68. While doing small movements?

Bei kleinen Bewegungen?

69. Were you in the hospital / in rehab?

Waren Sie im Krankenhaus /Kur?

70. For how long?
Wie lange?

71. Several days
MehrereTage

72. Several weeks
Mehrere Wochen

73. Several months
Mehrere Monate

74. When did you get discharged from the hospital?
Wann sind Sie vom Krankenhaus entlassen worden?

75. Yesterday
Gestern

76. The day before yesterday
Vorgestern

77. A few days ago

Vor ein Paar Tagen

78. How many?

Wieviele ?

79. A few weeks ago

Vor ein Paar Wochen

80. A few months ago

Vor ein Paar Monaten

Massage

Massage

1. Please get undressed

Ziehen Sie sich aus bitte

2. Can you please take off your top?

Können Sie Ihr Oberteil ausziehen?

3. Can you please take off your pants?

Können Sie Ihre Hose ausziehen?

4. Can you please take off your skirt?

Können Sie ihren Rock ausziehen?

5. Lie down on your back

Legen Sie sich auf den Rücken

6. Lie down on your stomach

Legen Sie sich auf den Bauch

7. Lie down on your right side

Legen Sie sich auf die rechte Seite

8. Lie down on your left side

Legen Sie sich auf die linke Seite

9. This is for your head

Kopf hier, bitte

10. Would you like a blanket?

Wollen Sie eine Decke?

11. Are you cold?

Ist Ihnen kalt ?

12. Are you too warm?

Ist Ihnen zu warm?

13. Put your right arm down

Legen Sie den rechten Arm runter

14. Put your right arm next to your head

Legen Sie den rechten Arm hoch

15. Align your right arm alongside your body

Legen Sie den rechten Arm am Körper entlang

16. Put your left arm down

Legen Sie den linken Arm runter

17. Put your left arm next to your head

Legen Sie den linken Arm hoch

18. Align your left arm alongside your body

Legen Sie den linken Arm am Körper entlang

19. Sit down please.

Setzen Sie sich hin, bitte

20. Relax your shoulders

Schulter locker lassen

21. Please look straigt ahead

Nach vorne schauen

22. Does it hurt?

Tut es weh?

23. Do I hurt you?

Tue ich Ihnen weh?

24. Show me where it hurts.

Zeigen Sie mir wo es weh tut

25. Is the pressure ok?

Ist der Druck gut?

26. Yes?

JA ?

27. No?

NEIN?

28. Harder?
   Stärker ?

29. Softer?
   Schwächer ?

30. Better?
   Besser?

31. Worse?
   Schlechter?

Manual therapy

Manuelle Therapie

1. **Please get undressed**
   Ziehen Sie sich aus bitte

2. **Can you please take off your top?**
   Können Sie Ihr Oberteil ausziehen?

3. **Can you please take off your pants?**
   Können Sie Ihre Hose ausziehen?

4. **Can you please take off your skirt?**
   Können Sie ihren Rock ausziehen?

5. **Where does it hurt?**
   Wo haben Sie Schmerzen?

6. **Has it improved since the last treatment?**
   Ist es besser geworden seit der letzten Behandlung?

7. Has it gotten worse?

Ist es schlechter geworden?

8. Has the pain increased?

Haben Sie jetzt mehr Schmerzen?

9. Has the pain gotten less?

Haben Sie jetzt weniger Schmerzen?

10. Where does it hurt now?

Wo sind jetzt die Schmerzen?

11. Stand on one leg please.

Stehen Sie auf ein Bein

12. Please stand on the other leg now.

Jetzt auf das andere Bein stehen

13. Stand on your heels

Stehen Sie auf die Fersen

14. Stand on your tiptoes

Stehen Sie auf die Fußspitzen

15. Sit down please
   Setzen Sie sich hin

16. Round your back
   Machen Sie sich rund

17. Put your chin to your chest
   Kopf einrollen

18. Does it pull?
   Zieht es?

19. Is it painful?
   Ist es schmerzhaft?

20. Is the pain less now?
   So weniger ?

21. Is the pain worse now?
   So mehr?

22. Better?
   Besser ?

23. Worse?

schlechter?

24. Put your head back

Heben Sie den Kopf

25. Lift your head up, look up

Kopf nach oben / nach oben schauen

26. Put your head down, look down

Kopf nach unten / nach unten schauen

27. Turn your head to the left

Kopf nach links drehen

28. Turn your head to the right

Kopf nach rechts drehen

29. Tilt your head to the left

Kopf nach links neigen

30. Tilt your head to the right

Kopf nach rechts neigen

31. Relax

Locker lassen

32. Do not help. I will do the movements, you relax

Nicht helfen, ich mache die Bewegung, Sie lassen locker

33. Put your arms up

Arme hoch

34. Put your right arm up

Rechter Arm hoch

35. Put your right arm down

Rechter Arm runter

36. Put your left arm up

Linker Arm hoch

37. Put your left arm down

Linker Arm runter

38. Bend your leg

Bein beugen

39. Extend your leg
Bein strecken

40. Bend your knee
Knie beugen

41. Extend your knee
Knie strecken

42. Lift your leg
Bein heben

43. Lie on your back
Legen Sie sich auf den Rücken

44. Lie on your stomach
Legen Sie sich auf den Bauch

45. Lie on your right side
Legen Sie sich auf die rechte Seite

46. Lie on your left side
Legen Sie sich auf die linke Seite

47. Put your head here, please

Kopf hier, bitte

48. Sit down

Setzen Sie sich hin

49. Please participate with ease

Machen Sie die Bewegung leicht mit.

50. Press against my resistance

Drücken Sie gegen meinen Widerstand

51. Press harder

Drücken Sie stärker

52. Press not so hard

Drücken Sie leichter

53. This is an exercise to do at home

Das ist eine Übung für Zuhause

54. Bend your legs and pull your knees to your thighs

Beine aufstellen

55. Tighten your Abdomen

Bauch anspannen

56. Squeeze your buttocks

Po anspannen

57. Tense your legs

Beine anspannen

58. Tense your arms

Arme anspannen

59. Relax

Entspannen

60. It might hurt a little

Es kann sein, dass es ein Bißchen weh tut

61. I will show you first, then you repeat

Ich zeige es Ihnen, dann machen Sie es nach

62. Do 3 sets with 10 repetitions

Machen Sie 3 Serien à 10 Wiederholungen

63. Do 3 sets with 15 repetitions
Machen Sie 3 Serien à 15 Wiederholungen

64. Do 3 sets with 20 repetitions
Machen Sie 3 Serien à 20 Wiederholungen

65. Do 3 sets with 30 repetitions
Machen Sie 3 Serien à 30 Wiederholungen

66. Once a week
1 mal die Woche

67. Twice a week
2 mal die Woche

68. Three times a week
3 mal die Woche

69. Once a day
1 mal pro Tag

70. Twice a day
2 mal pro Tag

71. Three times a day

3 mal pro Tag

72. Do the exercise in front of a mirror

Machen Sie die Übung vor dem Spiegel

73. Sit down in front of a mirror

Sitzen Sie vor dem Spiegel

74. Stand in front of a mirror

Stehen sie vor dem Spiegel

75. It is not supposed to hurt

Das darf nicht weh tun

76. This is not supposed to happen

Das darf nicht passieren

PNF

PNF

1. **Lie on your back**
   Legen Sie sich auf den Rücken

2. **Lie on your stomach**
   Legen Sie sich auf den Bauch

3. **Lie on your right side**
   Legen Sie sich auf die rechte Seite

4. **Lie on your left side**
   Legen Sie sich auf die linke Seite

5. **Put your head here, please**
   Kopf hier, bitte

6. **I will show you what the movement should look like**
   Ich zeige Ihnen wie die Bewegung aussehen soll

7. I will do the movement, relax your arm
   Ich mache die Bewegung, Sie lassen den Arm locker

8. I will do the movement, relax your leg
   Ich mache die Bewegung, Sie lassen das Bein locker

9. Press against my resistance now
   Jetzt drücken Sie gegen meinen Widerstand

10. Open your hand and extend your fingers
   Finger, Hand aufmachen

11. Close your hand aroung mine
   Finger, Hand zumachen

12. Extend your arm
   Ellbogen strecken

13. Bend your elbow
   Ellbogen beugen

14. Put your leg up
   Bein hoch

15. Put your leg down
Bein runter

16. Tense your leg in this direction
Bein in die Richtung anspannen

17. Bend your knee
Knie beugen

18. Extend your knee
Knie strecken

19. Bend your hips
Hüfte beugen

20. Extend your hips
Hüfte strecken

21. Relax
Entspannen / locker lassen

22. More
Mehr

23. Less
Weniger

24. Harder
Stärker

25. Softer
Schwächer

26. Slower
Langsamer

27. Faster
Schneller

28. Press upward
Nach oben drücken

29. Press downward
Nach unten drücken

30. Now in the other direction
Jetzt in die andere Richtung

31. Towards your opposite shoulder

Richtung gegenüberliegende Schulter

32. Towards your opposite hip

Richtung gegenüberliegende Hüfte

33. Towards the ear

Richtung Ohr

34. Towards the nose

Richtung Nase

35. Towards the window

Richtung Fenster

36. Towards the door

Richtung Tür

37. Towards the wall

Richtung Wand

38. Towards the clock

Richtung Uhr

Mulligan

Mulligan

1. Show me which movement causes the pain

Zeigen Sie mir bei welcher Bewegung sie Schmerzen haben

2. Relax

Lassen Sie locker

3. Repeat the movement once more

Machen Sie jetzt die Bewegung noch einmal

4. Is it better?

Ist es besser?

5. Do you have pain going upstairs?

Haben Sie Schmerzen bei Treppenhochsteigen ?

6. Do you have pain going downstairs?

Haben Sie Schmerzen bei Treppenruntersteigen ?

7. Is it better like this?

Ist es besser so?

8. You are not supposed to be in pain. Please say Stop if it hurts

Sie dürfen keine Schmerzen haben, wenn es weh tut sagen Sie Stopp.

9. If the strap hurts, I can put a pad between you and the strap

Wenn der Gurt weh tut lege ich ein Polster zwischen Ihnen und dem Gurt.

10. You can do this exercise with a towel at home

Daheim können Sie diese Übung mit einem Handtuch machen

11. you can do this exercise at home with an elastic band

Daheim können Sie diese Übung mit einem Theraband machen

12. You can do this exercise at home with a stick

Daheim können Sie diese Übung mit einem Stab machen

13. The ball can be purchased at a sporting goods store

Den Ball können Sie im Sportgeschäft kaufen.

14. The elastic band can be purchased at a sporting goods store

Das Theraband können Sie im Sportgeschäft kaufen.

15. It should be red

Es soll rot sein

16. It should be green

Es soll grün sein

Exercises

Übungen

1. **Bend**
   Beugen

2. **Extend**
   Strecken

3. **Flex**
   Anspannen

4. **Relax**
   Entspannen

5. **Move your buttocks backwards**
   Gesäß nach hinten

6. **tense your abdomen / do not relax**
   Bauch anspannen / angespannt lassen

7. Remain like this for a few seconds, then relax

Bleiben Sie so ein Paar Sekunden, dann entspannen

8. Do not move

Es darf keine Bewegung stattfinden

9. This is for your coordination

Das ist für die Koordination

10. Do 3 sets with 10 repetitions

Machen Sie 3 Serien à 10 Wiederholungen

11. Do 3 sets with 15 repetitions

Machen Sie 3 Serien à 15 Wiederholungen

12. Do 3 sets with 20 repetitions

Machen Sie 3 Serien à 20 Wiederholungen

13. Do 3 sets with 30 repetitions

Machen Sie 3 Serien à 30 Wiederholungen

14. Take a break between the sets

Machen Sie Pause zwischen den Serien

15. A few seconds

Ein Paar Sekunden

16. A few minutes

Ein Paar Minuten

17. How many

Wieviel?

18. Once a week

1 mal die Woche

19. Twice a week

2 mal die Woche

20. Three times a week

3 mal die Woche

21. Once a day

1 mal pro Tag

22. Twice a day

2 mal pro Tag

23. Three times a day
3 mal pro Tag

24. Do the exercise while standing in front of a mirror
Machen Sie die Übung vor dem Spiegel

25. Sit in front of the mirror
Sitzen Sie vor dem Spiegel

26. Stand in front of the mirror
Stehen sie vor dem Spiegel

27. This is for strengthening
Das ist für die Kräftigung

28. Do it at home every day
Zuhause jeden Tag machen

29. Do the exercises in front of the mirror so that you can correct yourself
Machen Sie die Übungen vor dem Spiegel damit Sie sich korrigieren können

30. This is not supposed to happen
Das darf nicht passieren

31. This is wrong
Das ist falsch

32. This is correct
So ist es richtig

33. Slow
Langsam

34. Slower
Langsamer

35. Fast
Schnell

36. Faster
Schneller

37. Don't jerk
Nicht ruckartig

38. Your are not supposed to be in pain during the exercise

Sie dürfen keine Schmerzen bei den Übungen haben.

39. If you are in pain doing the exercise please stop and tell me next time you are here.

Wenn Sie Schmerzen haben, während Sie die Übungen machen, lassen Sie die Übung sein und sagen es mir das nächste Mal.

40. Did you do the exercises?

Haben Sie die Übungen gemacht?

41. Did you feel any pain?

Haben Sie dabei Schmerzen gehabt?

42. Show me where it hurt?

Zeigen Sie mir wo Sie Schmerzen hatten

43. Show me how you do the exercises?

Zeigen Sie mir wie Sie die Übung machen.

44. Stand on your right leg
   Stehen sie auf dem rechten Bein

45. Stand on your left leg
   Stehen sie auf dem linken Bein

46. Stand on one leg
   Stehen sie auf einem Bein

47. This is for balance
   Das ist für das Gleichgewicht

48. Try not to move
   Versuchen Sie nicht zu wackeln

49. Try to include this exercise in your daily routine
   Diese Bewegung können Sie in den Alltag einbauen

Gait training

Gangschule

1. Stand straight
Stehen Sie gerade

2. Take smaller steps
Machen Sie kleinere Schritte

3. Take bigger steps
Machen Sie größere Schritte

4. Take regular steps
Machen Sie regelmäßige Schritte

5. Roll your foot from heel to toe
Den Fuß abrollen

6. First on your heel, roll your foot, then press your foot forward to your toes

Zuerst auf Ferse, dann rollt der Fuß, dann drücken Sie den Fuß vor mit dem Vorfuß

7. The crutch goes on the same side as your injured leg

Die Gehstütze gehen mit dem kranken Bein zusammen.

8. Swing your arms loosely by your body

Arme locker am Körper pendeln lassen

Lymphatic drainage

Lymphdrainage

1. The blood pressure cannot be taken on this arm nor can blood be drawn

An diesem Arm darf man kein Blutdruck messen oder Spritzen

2. Preferably you should not get hurt

Sie sollen sich möglichst nicht verletzten

3. You are not allowed to take a hot bath or lie in the sun for too long

Sie dürfen nicht heiß baden oder zu lange in der Sonne liegen

4. If you have a painful rash, see a doctor immediately

Wenn Sie einen schmerzhaften Ausschlag haben, gehen Sie sofort zum Arzt.

5. Put your legs up multiple times per day

Legen Sie oft, mehrmals pro Tag die Beine hoch

6. Put your leg up several times a day
   Legen Sie oft, mehrmals pro Tag das Bein hoch

7. Put your arm up multiple times a day
   Legen Sie oft, mehrmals pro Tag den Arm hoch

8. Do you have a surgical stocking?
   Haben Sie einen Kompressionsstrumpf ?

9. Do you have surgical stockings?
   Haben Sie Kompressionsstrümpfe?

10. You have to wear the stocking every day
   Den Strumpf müssen Sie jeden Tag tragen

11. You have to wear the stockings every day
   Die Strümpfe müssen Sie jeden Tag tragen

12. You have to wear the stocking night and day
   Den Strumpf müssen Sie Tag und Nacht tragen

13. You have to wear the stockings night and day
   Die Strümpfe müssen Sie Tag und Nacht tragen

14. You shouldn't wear tight-fitting clothes

Sie sollen keine einengende Kleidung tragen.

15. Lie on your back

Legen Sie sich auf den Rücken

16. Lie on your stomach

Drehen Sie sich auf den Bauch

17. Can you lie on your stomach or would your rather sit?

Können Sie sich auf den Bauch legen oder wollen Sie lieber sitzen?

18. Sit?

Sitzen?

19. Put one leg up

Bein aufstellen

20. Put both legs up

Beine aufstellen

21. Slide a little towards me

Ein Bisschen zu mir rutschen

22. Slide to the left

Rutschen Sie nach links

23. Slide to the right

Rutschen Sie nach rechts

24. Slide up

Rutschen Sie kopfwärts

25. Slide down

Rutschen Sie fußwärts

26. Does it hurt?

Tut es weh?

27. It shouldn't hurt

Es darf nicht weh tun

Electrotherapy

Elektrotherapie

1. I will attach 2 electrodes

Ich werde 2 Elektroden anlegen

2. I will attach 4 electrodes

Ich werde 4 Elektroden anlegen

3. There is no electricity yet

Es fließt noch kein Strom

4. I will increase the electricity slowly

Ich drehe den Strom langsam hoch

5. Tell me, as soon as you feel the electricity

Sie sagen es mir sobald Sie Strom spüren

6. Do you feel the electricity?

Spüren Sie den Strom?

7. It should be comfortable

Es soll angenehm sein

8. Is it comfortable?

Ist es angenehm?

9. You should feel the electricity only slightly

Sie sollen den Strom nur ganz leicht spüren

10. I will turn down the electricity until you can't feel it anymore

Jetzt drehe ich den Strom runter bis Sie ihn nicht mehr spüren

11. It will take about 10 minutes

Es dauert circa 10 Minuten

12. It will take about 15 minutes

Es dauert circa 15 Minuten

13. It will take about 20 minutes

Es dauert circa 20 Minuten

14. I will take off the electrodes once it is finished

Wenn es fertig ist, komme ich und mache die Elektroden weg.

15. If you have a problem, call me

Wenn Sie ein Problem haben, rufen Sie mich.

16. I will be next-door

Ich bin nebenan

pelvic floor exercises

Beckenboden Gymnastik

short

1. The pelvic floor is the muscle between your pubic bone and your tailbone

Der Beckenboden ist der Muskel der zwischen Schambein und Steißbein ist.

2. Its function is mainly to close the openings there

Seine Aufgabe ist hauptsächlich die Öffnungen, die sich da befinden zu schließen.

3. It works together with you abdominal muscles and your diaphragm

Er arbeitet mit den Bauchmuskeln und mit dem Zwerchfell zusammen.

4. In order to strengthen your pelvic floor you have to use these muscles as well

Deshalb muß man diese Muskeln auch mitarbeiten lassen um den Beckenboden zu kräftigen.

5. **Try to tense your pelvic floor, acting like have to use the bathroom but you can't go**

   Versuchen Sie den Beckenboden anzuspannen indem Sie so anspannen wie wenn Sie aufs Klo müssten, es aber nicht könnten.

<u>**Long**</u>

1. **The pelvic floor is the muscle between ischial tuberosities, pubic and tailbone**

   Der Beckenboden ist der Muskel der sich zwischen rechter und linker Sitzbeinhöcker, Steißbein und Schambein befindet. Durch regelmäßiges Training können Sie einer Inkontinenz vorbeugen oder bestehende Probleme günstig beeinflussen.

2. **The pelvic floor helps to control the function of urinating and bowel movement. With regular training you can prevent incontinence or lessen exiting problems**

   Der Beckenboden trägt wesentlich dazu bei, dass Sie Ihren Urin- und Stuhlabgang kontrollieren können.

3. **In addition, the pelvic floor holds and supports the organs in your abdomen. That's why regular pelvic floor training works against prolapse problems**

   Weiterhin bietet der Beckenboden den inneren Bauchorganen Halt und stützt sie von unten. Daher können Sie mit einem Becken-bodentraining Senkungsbeschwerden entgegenwirken.

4. **To fulfill these functions, the pelvic floor works with the abdominal muscles and the diaphragm, which is the most important respiratory muscle.**

   Um diese Aufgaben erfüllen zu können, arbeitet der Beckenboden zusammen mit der Bauchmuskulatur und dem Zwerchfell, dem wichtigsten Atemmuskel.

5. **In order to strengthen your pelvic floor you have to use these muscles as well**

   Deshalb muß man diese Muskeln auch mitarbeiten lassen um den Beckenboden zu kräftigen.

6. **Try to tighten your pelvic floor, imagining closing your vagina and anus**

   Versuchen Sie, die Beckenbodenmuskulatur anzuspannen indem Sie sich vorstellen daß Sie Ihren After und Ihre Scheide verschließen.

7. Try to tighten your pelvic floor, acting like have to use the toilet but you can't go

Versuchen Sie den Beckenboden anzuspannen indem Sie so anspannen wie wenn Sie aufs Klo müssten, es aber nicht könnten.

8. Inhale deeply. Exhale slowly tensing your abdominal muscles

Tief einatmen, beim langsamen Ausatmen Bauch anspannen.

9. I will show you, and then you do it

Ich zeige es Ihnen, dann machen Sie es nach.

Breathing therapy

Atemtherapie

1. Inhale through your nose

Atmen Sie durch die Nase ein

2. Exhale through your mouth

Atmen Sie durch den Mund aus

3. I will show you, and then you do it

Ich mache es vor, Sie machen es nach.

4. Slowly

Langsam

5. Slower

Langsamer

6. Fast

Schnell

7. Faster
Schneller

8. Deeply
Tief

9. Deeper
Tiefer

10. Casual
Oberflächig

11. More casually
Oberflächiger

12. Inhale more into your abdomen
Atmen Sie mehr in den Bauch

13. Your abdomen should expand when inhaling
Der Bauch soll dicker werden wenn Sie einatmen.

14. Put your hands on your abdomen

Legen Sie die Hände auf den Bauch

15. Put your hands on your ribcage

Legen Sie die Hände auf den Brustkorb

16. Your hands should be moving on your abdomen when inhaling

Ihre Hände sollen vom Bauch bewegt werden wenn Sie einatmen

Useful

Nützliches

1. Hello
Guten Tag

2. Goodbye
Tschüss

3. Please
Bitte

4. Thank you
Danke

5. Relax
Locker lassen

6. Does it hurt?
Tut es weh?

7. Is it better now?
 Ist es besser so?

8. Harder?
 Stärker?

9. Yes
 Ja

10. No
 Nein

11. I'm sorry, I can't understand you
 Es tut mir Leid, ich verstehe Sie nicht

Thanks

I would like to thank all those who helped me to create the Little Physio book and application.

Thanks to the translators and the proof-readers, thanks to my family and my friends who have all participated in this adventure.

Thanks to those who helped with their voice on the apps and the videos.

Special thanks to my husband who programmed the apps for android and apple and for everything else too... :)

Thank you, dear reader for having bought this book or any of my other books.

If you have enjoyed Little Physio,
please leave comments on Amazon.

I would appreciate it very much :)

Bibliography

- **Little Physio** from English into Spanish
- **Little Physio** from English into Italian
- **Little Physio** from English into French
- **Little Physio** from English into German
- **Little Physio** from English into Turkish

and

- **Big Little Physio** from English into Spanish, Italian, French, German and Turkish

www.ingramcontent.com/pod-product-compliance
Lightning Source LLC
Chambersburg PA
CBHW071802170526
45167CB00003B/1134